Counting
Calories

ISBN: 1 86476 103 2

This edition for
SELECT EDITIONS
Devizes
Wiltshire, UK

The images used in this book are from IMSI's Masterclips Collection,
75 Rowland Way, Novato, CA 94945, USA.

Counting
Calories

Contents

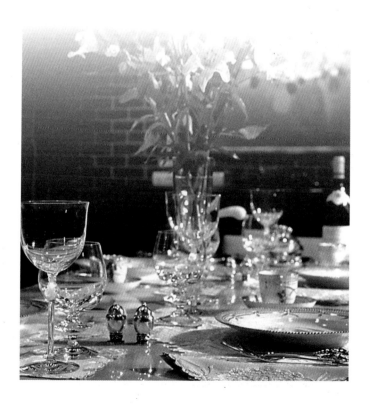

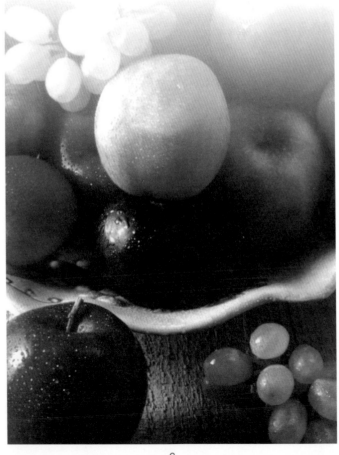

Fruit

Fruit: per 100g	Cal	Fat
Apple, raw, with core	42	0.1
Apple, raw, peeled	45	0.1
Apricots, canned in natural juice	34	0.1
Apricots, canned in syrup	63	0.1
Apricot	31	0.1
Avocado	190	19.5
Banana	95	0.3
Blackberries	62	0.2
Blackcurrants, canned in natural juice	31	1.0
Blackcurrants, canned in syrup	71	1.0
Blackcurrants, raw	28	1.0
Cantaloupe	19	0.1
Cherries in syrup	71	1.0
Cherries, glace	251	1.0
Cherries, raw	48	0.1
Currants	264	0.4
Dates, dried	227	0.2
Dates, raw	107	0.1
Figs, dried	227	1.6

Figs, semi dried	209	1.5
Fruit Salad, canned in natural juice	29	1.0
Fruit Salad, canned in syrup	57	1.0
Grapefruit, canned in natural juice	30	1.0
Grapefruit, canned in syrup	60	1.0
Grapefruit, raw	20	0.1
Honeydew	28	0.1
Grapes	60	0.1
Kiwi Fruit	49	0.5
Lemons	19	0.3
Mandarins	32	1.0
Mangoes, canned in syrup	77	1.0
Mangoes, raw	57	0.2
Nectarines	40	0.1
Olives, in brine	103	11.0
Oranges	37	0.1
Paw-paw	36	0.1
Peaches, canned in natural juice	39	1.0
Peaches, canned in syrup	50	1.0
Peaches, raw	40	0.1
Peel, mixed	231	0.9
Pineapple, canned in natural juice	47	1.0

Pineapple, canned in syrup	64	1.0
Pineapple, raw	41	0.2
Plums, canned in syrup	59	1.0
Plums, raw	34	0.1
Prunes, canned in natural juice	79	0.2
Prunes, canned in syrup	90	0.2
Prunes, semi dried	141	0.2
Raisins	272	0.4
Raspberries, canned in syrup	31	1.0
Raspberry, raw	25	0.3
Rhubarb, canned in syrup	65	1.0
Rhubarb, raw	7	0.1
Strawberries	27	0.1
Sultanas	275	0.4
Tangerines	35	0.1
Watermelon	31	0.3

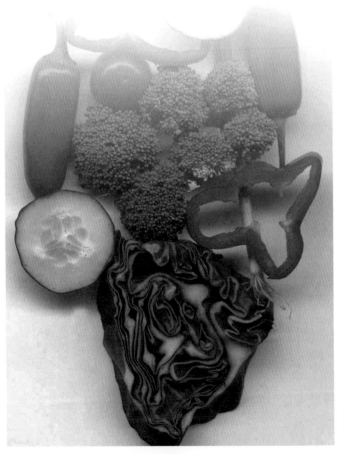

Vegetables

Vegetables: per 100g	Cal	Fat
Alfalfa/Bean Sprouts	30	0
Asparagus, raw	25	0.6
Aubergine	15	0.4
Bamboo Shoots, canned, drained	39	0
Baked Beans in tom sauce	84	0.6
Broad Beans	81	0.6
Butter Beans, canned	77	0.5
French Beans	25	0.1
Red Kidney Beans, canned	100	0.6
Red Kidney Beans, dried	103	0.5
Runner Beans	22	0.4
Soya Beans, dried	141	7.3
Beetroot, raw	36	0.1
Broccoli	33	0.9
Brussel Sprouts,	42	1.4
Cabbage	26	0.4
Carrots	34	0.9
Celery	7	0.2
Chick Peas, canned	115	2.9

Chick Peas, dried	121	2.1
Cucumber	10	0.1
Fennel	12	0.2
Garlic	98	0.6
Gherkins, pickled	14	0.1
Humus	187	12.6
Leeks	22	0.5
Lentils, dried	105	0.7
Lettuce	14	0.5
Marrow	12	0.2
Mushrooms	135	0.5
Okra	31	1.0
Onions, pickled	24	0.2
Onion, raw	36	0.2
Parsnip	64	1.1
Peas, boiled	79	1.6
Peas, canned	80	0.9
Plantain	117	0.3
Potatoes	70	0
Potatoes, mashed with butter & milk	100	3.0
Potatoes, roasted in fat	125	5.5
Potato Chips – straight cut	200	7.0
Potato Chips – Crinkle cut	240	10

Potato Chips – French Fries	290	15
Potato Chips – Oven Fried	210	10
Pumpkin	13	0.2
Radish	12	0.2
Spinach	25	0.8
Split Peas, dry	300	2.0
Split Peas, cooked	60	0.5
Spring Onions	23	0.5
Swede	24	0.3
Sweet Potato	84	0.3
Sweetcorn, baby, canned	23	0.4
Sweetcorn, kernels, canned	122	1.2
Sweetcorn, on the cob	66	1.4
Tofu – Soya bean, steamed	73	4.2
Tomato Puree	68	0.2
Tomatoes, canned with juice	16	0.1
Tomatoes, grilled	49	0.9
Tomatoes, raw	17	0.3
Turnip	12	0.2
Watercress	22	1.0
Yam	100	

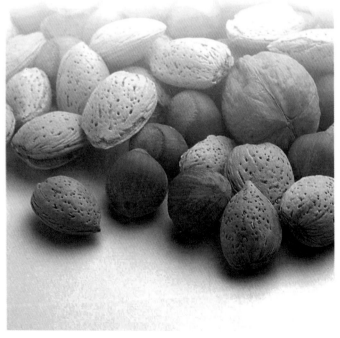

Nuts & Seeds

Nuts: per 100g	Cal	Fat
Almonds	612	55.8
Brazil Nuts	682	68.2
Cashew Nuts, roasted, salted	611	50.9
Chestnuts	170	2.7
Coconut, creamed	669	68.8
Coconut, dessicated	604	62.0
Hazelnuts	650	63.5
Macadamia Nuts	748	77.6
Mixed Nuts	607	54.1
Peanuts, plain	564	46.1
Peanuts, roasted, salted	602	53.0
Peanuts, dry, roasted	589	49.8
Pecan Nuts	689	70.1
Pistachio Nuts	331	30.5
Walnuts	688	68.5
Nut based Products: per 100g		
Marzipan	404	14.4
Peanut Butter	623	53.7
Seeds: per 100g		
Sesame seeds	579	58.0
Sunflower seeds	581	47.5

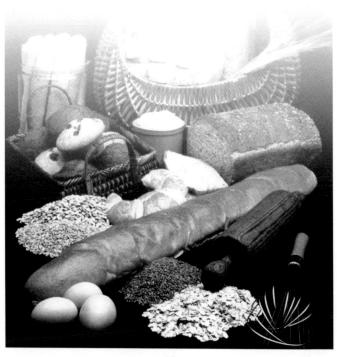

Bread & Cereal Products

Biscuits: per 100g	Cal	Fat
Cheddars	534	30.2
Cheeselets	464	21.7
Chocolate, assorted	524	27.6
Chocolate, mint	521	30.0
Double Choc	539	29.8
Digestive	499	22.1
Gingernut	456	15.2
Semi-sweet	457	16.6
Short-sweet	469	23.4
Wafer filled	535	29.9
Oatcakes	441	18.3
Shortbread	498	26.1
Bread: per 100g		
Brown bread, average	218	2.0
Croissants	360	20.3
Crumpets	199	1.0
Hamburger bun	264	5.0
Hot Cross Buns	310	6.8
Malt bread	268	2.4

Naan bread	336	12.5
Pitta bread	265	1.2
Roll, brown	255	2.8
Roll, white	280	2.3
Roll, wholemeal	241	2.9
Rye bread	219	1.7
White bread, with added fibre	230	1.5
White bread, average	235	1.9
White, french stick	270	2.7
Wholemeal. Average	215	2.5
Breakfast Cereal: per 100g		
All-bran	261	3.4
Bran Flakes	318	1.9
Coco Pops	384	1.0
Corn Flakes	360	0.7
Crunchy Nut Corn Flakes	398	4.0
Frosties	377	0.5
Muesli	366	7.8
Porridge, with milk	116	5.1
Porridge, with water	49	1.1
Puffed Wheat	321	1.3
Special K	377	1.0

Sultana Bran	303	1.6
Rice : per 100g		
Brown rice	358	2.5
Brown & White blend	356	2.5
White rice	354	0.5
Wild rice	358	2.5
Crackers: per 100g		
Wholemeal	413	11.3
Rye	321	2.1
Custard powder: per 100g		
Custard powder	354	0.7
Flour: per 100g		
Cornflour	354	0.7
Rye flour	335	2.0
Soya, full fat	447	23.5
Soya, low fat	352	7.2
Wheat, brown	232	1.8
Wheat, white, plain	341	1.3
Wheat, white, self-raising	330	1.2
Wheat, wholemeal	310	2.2
Noodles: per 100g		
Dry, average	350	1.0

Egg noodles, raw	391	8.2
Egg noodles, boiled	62	0.5
Pasta: per 100g		
Shells/Spirals, dry	345	1.0
Guzzis, dry	345	1.5
Macaroni	348	1.8
Macaroni cheese	178	10.8
Ravioli, canned in tomato sauce	70	2.2
Spaghetti, canned in tomato sauce	64	0.4
Spaghetti	342	1.8
Spaghetti, wholemeal	324	2.5
Wholemeal/Vege	320	2.0
Kid's pasta	370	2.0

Eggs & Egg Based Dishes

Chicken Eggs: per 100g	Cal	Fat
Boiled	147	10.8
Fried in vegetable oil	179	13.9
Scrambled with milk	247	22.6
White (raw)	36	1.0
Yolk (raw)	339	30.5
Omelette, cheese	266	22.6
Omelette, plain	191	16.4
Quiche, cheese & egg	314	22.2

Fresh Milk

Full Cream: per 100g	Cal	Fat
Regular	151	9.4
Reduced Fat: per 250ml		
Skimmer	118	4.0
Skim/Non fat milk: per 250ml		
Regular	88	0.5
Longlife: per 250ml		
Full Cream (average all brands)	167	9.5
Reduced Fat	145	5.0
Skim/Nonfat	87	0.5
Lactose Reduced	170	1.0
Soy Milk Drinks: per 100g		
Plain (average)	32	1.9
Flavoured (average)	40	1.7
Flavoured Milk: per 100g		
Milk Shake (average)	350	12
Thick Shake (average)	275	10
Smoothie (average)	300	10
Flavoured Milk (average) per 100g	243	11
Flavoured Milk – skimmer (average) per 100g	68	1.5

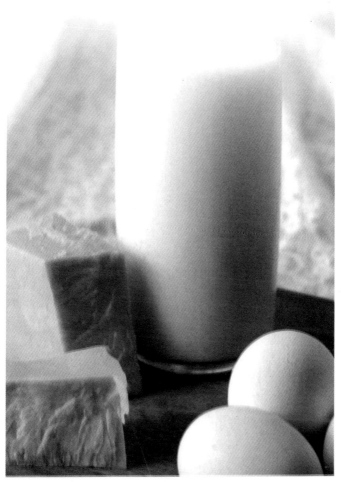

Yogurt

Average all brands: per 100g	Cal	Fat
Low Fat (flavoured)	90	0.9
Low Fat (with fruit)	90	0.7
Plain (Natural)	80	2.5
Plain (Non-fat/Skim)	60	0.2
Frozen Yogurt (all flavours)		

Cheese

Average all brands: per 100g	Cal	Fat
Brie	319	26.9
Camembert	297	23.7
Cheddar	412	34.4
Cheddar (vegetarian)	425	35.7
Cheddar (reduced fat)	261	15.0
Cheese spread	276	22.8
Cottage Cheese	98	3.9
Cottage Cheese (reduced fat)	78	1.4
Cottage Cheese (with additions)	95	3.8
Cream Cheese	439	47.4
Cream Cheese (reduced fat)	285	22.5
Danish Blue	347	29.6
Edam	333	25.4
Feta	250	20.2
Fromage (with fruit)	131	5.8
Fromage (plain)	113	7.1
Fromage (low fat)	58	0.2
Gouda	375	31.0
Hard Cheese	405	34.0
Parmesan	452	32.7
Soft Cheese	313	31.0

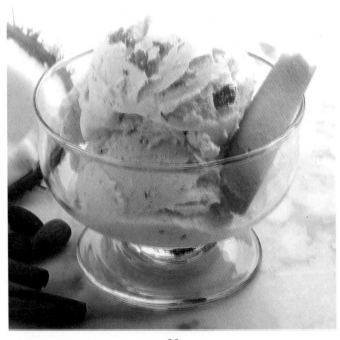

Ice Cream

Average all brands: per 100g	Cal	Fat
Choc Ice	277	17.5
Cornetto	260	12.9
Flavoured	8.0	179
Vanilla	180	10
Vanilla, low fat	140	4.0
Vanilla, reduced fat	170	6.0
Super Premium: per 100g		
e.g. Connoisseur, Sara Lee	250	1.0

Cream

Average: per 20g	Cal	Fat
Sour Cream (per 20g)	38	3.5
Sour Cream light (per 20g)	28	3.0
Thickened Cream (per 20g)	67	7.0
Whipping Cream (per 20g)	160	12.0
Double Cream (per 20g)	115	11.0

Meat

Steak: per 100g	Cal	Fat
Blade Steak (lean, grilled)	175	7.0
Corned Beef (lean+ fat, cooked)	245	14
Corned Beef (lean only, cooked)	210	9.5
Chuck Steak (lean+ fat, cooked)	122	4.5
Chuck Steak (lean only, cooked)	108	3.0
Fillet Steak (lean+ fat, grilled)	206	9.5
Fillet Steak (lean, grilled)	196	8.5
Rib Steak (lean+ fat, grilled)	215	11.0
Rib Steak (lean only, grilled)	176	6.0
Ribeye Steak (lean +fat, grilled)	215	10
Ribeye Steak (lean only, grilled)	197	8.0
Round Steak (lean+ fat, grilled)	183	7.0
Round Steak (lean only, grilled)	176	6.0
Rump Steak (lean+ fat, grilled)	213	10
Rump Steak (lean only, grilled)	190	7.0
Roast Beef (lean+ fat, roasted)	160	6.5
Roast Beef (lean only, roasted)	150	5.0
Silverside Roast (lean+ fat, roasted)	192	6.5
Silverside Roast (lean only, roasted)	177	4.5

Sirloin Steak (lean+ fat, grilled)	216	12.0
Sirloin Steak (lean only, grilled)	192	9.0
T-Bone Steak (lean+ fat, grilled)	165	8.0
T-Bone Steak (lean only, grilled)	135	5.5
Topside Strips (raw)	125	4.0
Topside Strips (Stir fried)	163	6.5
Mince: per 100g		
Hamburger mince – 80% fat free	250	25.0
Steak mince – 90% fat free	170	10.0
Steak mince (cooked)	170	9.0
Lamb: per 100g		
Roast leg of lamb (lean+ fat, roasted)	190	7.5
Roast leg of lamb (lean, roasted)	175	5.5
Lamb Strips (raw)	135	6.0
Lamb Steak (topside, raw)	131	6.0
Lamb Steak (topside, raw)	127	4.5
Loin Chop (raw)	200	14.0
Loin Chop (grilled)	170	10.0
Butterfly Steak (raw)	172	10.0
Eye of Loin (raw)	119	5.0
Lamb fillet (raw)	138	6.5

Veal: per 100g

Forequarter (lean+ fat, cooked)	155	4.5
Forequarter (lean only, cooked)	134	2.5
Leg Roast (lean+ fat, roasted)	140	1.5
Leg Roast (lean only, roasted)	132	1.0
Schnitzel Steak (fried, 77g)	75	2.0
Schnitzel Steak (crumbed & pan fried – 180g)	309	25.0
Veal Shank (raw)	50	1.0

Pork: per 100g

Forequarter Chop (lean+ fat, grilled)	225	16.0
Forequarter Chop (lean only, grilled)	162	6.5
Forequarter Roast (lean+ fat, roasted)	215	14.0
Forequarter Roast (lean only, roasted)	157	6.5
Spare Ribs (lean with fat)	115	9.0
Pork mince (raw)	315	28.0

New Fashioned Pork: per 100g

Loin Chop (lean+ fat, grilled)	180	10.0
Loin Chop (lean only, grilled)	145	4.0
Leg Steak (lean+ fat, grilled)	140	3.0
Leg Steak (lean only, grilled)	125	1.5
Leg Schnitzel (lean+ fat, pan fried)	147	3.5

Leg Schnitzel (lean only, pan fried)	134	1.5
Leg Strips (lean+ fat, stir fried)	142	3.0
Leg Strips (lean only, stir fried)	134	1.5
Butterfly Steak (lean+ fat, grilled)	190	7.5
Butterfly Steak (lean only, grilled)	157	3.0
Pork Fillet (lean+ fat, grilled)	134	3.0
Pork Fillet (lean only, grilled)	122	2.0
Pork mince (raw)	143	7.0
Pork mince (cooked)	186	9.0
Bacon		
Middle rashers – 50g (lean+ fat, fried)	112	9.0
Middle rashers – 50g (lean+ fat, grilled)	97	7.0
Game: per 100g		
Buffalo (lean, cooked)	155	1.0
Camel (raw)	100	2.0
Crocodile (raw)	120	4.0
Emu (lean, grilled)	150	3.0
Goat (roasted)	150	3.0
Kangaroo (lean, raw)	150	1.0
Pigeon (roasted)	230	13.0
Rabbit (raw)	125	4.0
Venison (lean+ fat)	200	6.0

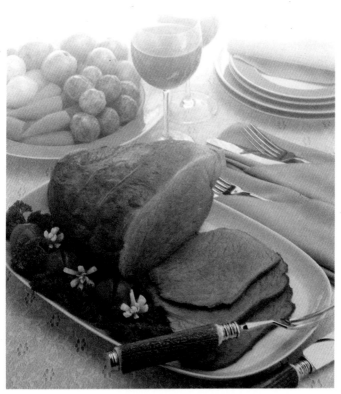

Chicken & Turkey

Roasted or Rotisseried	Cal	Fat
Breast – small (with skin)	310	18.0
Breast – small (no skin)	185	5.0
Breast – medium (with skin)	420	25.0
Breast – medium (no skin)	250	8.0
Breast – large (with skin)	485	29.0
Breast – large (no skin)	290	9.0
Drumstick – small (with skin)	100	6.0
Drumstick – small (no skin)	65	3.0
Drumstick – large (with skin)	120	8.0
Drumstick – large (no skin)	85	4.0
Thigh – small (with skin)	185	12.0
Thigh – small (no skin)	125	6.0
Thigh – Large (with skin)	225	14.0
Thigh – Large (no skin)	165	8.0
Wing – small (with skin)	70	5.0
Wing – small (no skin)	20	1.0
Wing – large (with skin)	100	7.0
Wing – large (no skin)	40	2.0

Chicken Products: per 100g

Chicken Drumsticks	117	5.0
Chicken Thighs (with skin)	182	13.0
Chicken Wings (with skin)	180	12.0
Chicken fillet – Breast (with skin)	130	5.0
Chicken fillet – Breast (no skin)	96	1.0
Chicken fillet – Thigh (with skin)	146	8.0
Chicken fillet – Thigh (no skin)	127	6.0
Chicken fillet – Maryland (with skin)	150	8.5
Chicken fillet – Maryland (no skin)	132	6.0

Turkey: per 100g

Meat & skin (raw, with skin)	145	7.0
Meat & skin (raw, no skin)	110	2.0
Roasted Turkey (with skin)	170	6.5
Roasted Turkey (no skin)	140	3.0
Light meat (lean, no skin)	130	1.5
Dark meat (lean, no skin)	150	4.0

Sausages: Beef, Pork Mutton

Thin sausages 70g (raw)	180	15.0
Thin sausages 70g (cooked)	155	12.0

Thick sausages 100g (raw)	260	22.0
Thick sausages 100g (cooked)	200	15.0
Reduced fat 70g (raw)	140	11.0
Reduced fat 70g (cooked)	120	9.0
Low fat sausages 70g (raw)	105	6.0
Low fat sausages 70g (cooked)	95	5.0
Cocktail Frankfurts 25g each	60	5.0
Canned Frankfurts 50g each	96	7.5
Saveloys (raw, 75g)	210	17.0
Saveloys (cooked 75g)	170	13.0

Lunch Meats: per 100g

Berliner fleischer	226	18.2
Brawn	153	11.5
Chicken Roll	151	9.3
Devon chicken, devon ham & chicken	234	18.5
Garlic roll	246	18.9
Liverwurst	276	28.8
Mortadella	324	29.3
Polish sausage	240	17.8
Salami – average all varieties	427	37.6
Strasbourg	245	19.2

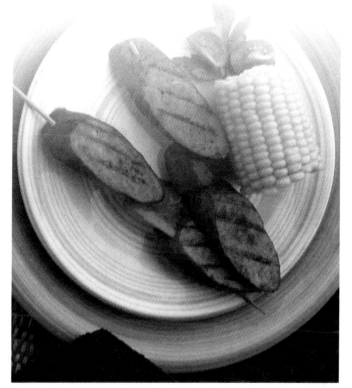

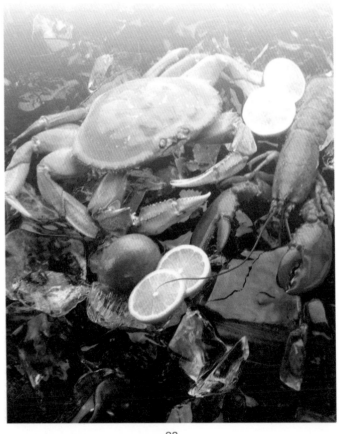

Fish & Shellfish

Fish & Shellfish: per 100g	Cal	Fat
Abalone (raw)	105	0.5
Anchovies (flat)	180	8.9
Barramundi (raw)	86	1.0
Bream (steamed)	139	3.7
Calamari	80	1.0
Caviar – black (1 tsp, 19g)	17	1.0
Caviar – red (1 tsp, 19g)	29	1.6
Clams (meat only)	80	1.0
Cockles (boiled)	48	0.5
Coral Trout (raw)	90	1.0
Crab (cooked)	100	2.0
Crayfish/Lobster	90	1.0
Eel (raw)	185	12.0
Mackerel (raw)	100	1.0
Mussels (shelled, raw)	90	2.0
Octopus (raw)	75	1.0
Oysters (shelled, raw, 60g)	40	1.5
Prawns/Shrimp (boiled)	107	2.0

Salmon/Tuna Patty (medium, 50g)	120	12.0
Schnapper (raw)	90	0.5
Swordfish (raw)	120	4.0
Trout, Rainbow (raw)	120	2.5
Frozen Fish		
Average all brands:		
Fish Fingers 25g	50	3.0
Fish Cakes 50g	100	5.5
Fish Fillets 100g	80	0.5
Fish Fillets (fried, 100g)	275	18.0
Prawns (cooked & peeled 100g)	107	2.0
Crab/Seafood Stick 30g	30	0.5
Seafood Extender 30g	25	0.5
Canned Fish		
Average all brands:		
Anchovies (drained 30g)	65	4.5
Caviar (Cod Roe,15g)	40	3.0
Clams 100g	85	2.0
Crabmeat 100g	100	1.0
Herrings in Tomato sauce 100g	190	11.0
Kipper Fillets 100g	220	18.0

Oysters/Mussels (drained, 100g)	200	12.0
Salmon – Pink, 100g	135	6.0
Salmon – Red, 100g	175	11.0
Sardines 100g	300	26.0
Shrimps (drained, 100g)	94	1.5
Tuna (brine/water, 100g)	105	2.0
Tuna (oil, 100g)	265	23.0
Fish spreads/Pastes	45	3.0

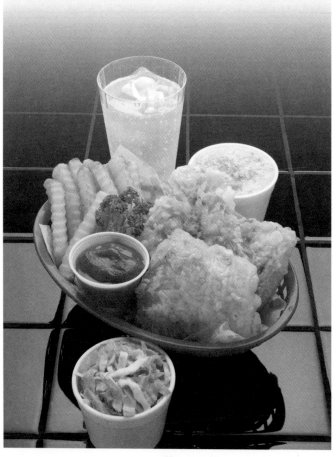

Take Away

Hungry Jacks	Cal	Fat
Bacon Double Cheeseburger	650	40.0
Bacon Double Cheeseburger Deluxe	710	48.0
Cheese Burger	390	20.0
Grilled Chicken Burger	410	20.0
Junior Whopper with cheese	460	28.0
Ocean Catch	400	17.0
Whopper	660	39.0
Whopper with cheese	750	46.0
Whopper with bacon	705	42.0
Whopper with egg	690	40.0
French fries – small	230	12.0
French fries – large	470	25.0
Strawberry sundae	220	7.0
Chocolate, Caramel sundae	240	9.0

KFC

Drumstick	140	8.0
Wing	130	10.0
Breast	250	15.0
Rib	230	15.0
Thigh	290	22.0
Nuggets – 6 pack	300	17.0
Chicken fillet burger	300	17.0
Bacon & Cheese chicken fillet burger	460	22.0
Works Chicken fillet burger	500	23.0
Zinger Burger	425	17.0
Bacon & Cheese/Works Burger	490	18.0
Crispy Strips – 3 pieces	260	16.0
Chips – Regular 120g	330	20.0
Chips – Large 230g	645	40.0
Potato & Gravy 120g	80	2.0

McDonalds

Big Mac	495	24.0
Cheese Burger	315	12.0

Double Cheeseburger	430	22.0
Filet-O-Fish	370	16.0
Junior Burger	270	8.0
McChicken Burger	470	22.0
Quarter Pounder	460	20.0
Quarter Pounder with cheese	560	28.0
Nuggets – 6 pack	305	18.0
French fries – small	285	16.0
French fries – large	525	29.0
Big Breakfast	572	32.0
Bacon & Egg McMuffin	342	17.0
English Muffin	157	3.5
Hash Brown	155	10.0
Hot Cakes with butter & syrup	440	9.0
Sausage McMuffin with egg	300	15.0
Apple Pie	260	15.0
Hot fudge sundae	320	11.0
Hot caramel sundae	315	8.0
Strawberry sundae	255	6.0

Frozen and packaged foods:

Pies: Average all brands

Family Pie 125g	320	18.0
Meat/Pork pie 170g	400	23.0
Party Pies 43g	120	8.0

Sausage Rolls: Average all brands

Small/Party	90	5.0
Medium/Regular	210	11.0
Large	270	14.0

Beef/Hamburger Patty: Average all brands

1 patty (grilled, 50g)	100	7.0
1 patty (fried, 50g)	110	8.5

Frozen Pizza: Average all brands

1/2 large 125g	275	9.0
1 large 500g	1095	36.0
Singles/snacks 100g	240	9.0

Lean Cuisine: per pack

Chicken Marsala	195	5.0
Creamy Vegetable Bake	240	7.5
Oriental Beef	270	6.0

Traditional Lasagne	265	5.5
Tuna Lasagne	310	7.5
Larger serves		
Lean Beef Lasagne 400g	440	8.5
Satay Lamb 400g	490	12.0
Thai Chicken Curry 400g	440	12.0
Vegetable Lasagne 400g	420	6.0
Maggi		
Beef Stroganoff 380g	407	7.0
Chicken in Apricot 355g	447	13.0
Lasagne 400g	430	10.0
Rich Gravy Beef	312	9.5
Shepherd's Pie 460g	470	19.0
Spaghetti Bolognaise 400g	402	13.0
Tomato & Onion Sausages 390g	470	26.0
Tuna Mornay 400g	402	14.0
McCain: Healthy Choice, per pack		
Beef in Black Bean Sauce	292	4.0
Chicken Chasseur	252	3.5
Honey Sesame Chicken	300	5.5

Pepper Steak	280	8.0
Roast Pork	300	3.5
Satay Beef	300	6.0
Tandoori Chicken	300	5.5
Vegetarian Lasagne	300	7.0
Larger sizes		
Chicken Teriyaki with rice	487	10.0
Creamy Chicken Carbonara	485	12.0
Stirfry Beef & Noodles	484	9.0
Stirfry Chicken & Noodles	460	9.0
Red Box		
Beef Hot Pot	357	11.0
Beef Stroganoff	460	15.0
Chicken Parmigiana	428	17.0
Fried Rice	475	9.0
Fettucine Carbonara	555	31.0
Lasagne	542	24.0
Roast Beef	240	4.0
Roast Chicken	315	9.5

Roast Lamb	286	7.0
Roast Pork	278	5.5
Roast Turkey	264	3.5
Shepherds Pie	415	18.0
Spaghetti Bolognaise	483	12.0
Steak Diane	322	12.0
Sweet & Sour Chicken	348	4.0
Tuna Mornay	627	28.0

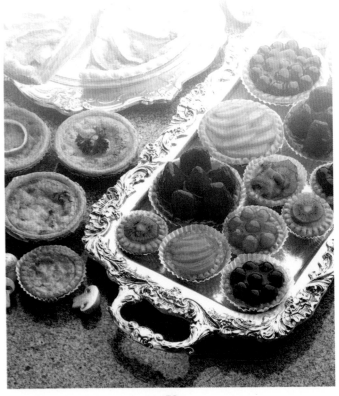

Sweets & Savories

Chocolate: per 100g	Cal	Fat
Aero Bar	522	28.7
Bounty Bar	473	26.1
Chocolate Cream	425	13.7
Chocolate, milk	529	30.3
Chocolate, plain	525	29.2
Chocolate, white	529	30.9
Chocolate, filled, assorted	460	18.8
Crème egg	385	16.8
Crunchie	460	19.1
Dairy Milk	525	29.4
Flake	505	28.5
Fudge	420	17.2
Kit Kat	499	26.6
Mars Bar	441	18.9
Milky Way	397	15.8
Smarties	456	17.5
Toblerone	530	31.0
Turkish Delight	370	7.7
Twirl	525	30.1

Twix	480	24.5
Violet Crumble	460	18.0
Confectionery: per 100g		
Boiled sweets	327	1.0
Fruit Gums	172	0
Liquorice Allsorts	313	2.2
Peppermints	392	0.7
Toffees, mixed	430	17.2
Cakes: per 100g		
Black Forest Cake	330	18.0
Cake muffins	280	13.0
Carrot Cake with Icing	375	10.0
Doughnut, iced	397	21.7
Doughnut, jam	336	14.5
Éclair	396	30.6
Gateau	337	16.8
Mud Cake	350	16.0
Scones, fruit	316	9.8
Scones, plain	362	14.6
Scones, wholemeal	326	11.7

Sponge, basic	459	26.3
Sponge, low fat	294	6.1
Sponge, jam filled	302	4.9
Sponge, butter icing	490	30.6
Swiss Rolls, chocolate	337	11.3
Teacakes	329	8.3
Savories: per 100g		
Corn Chips	490	23.0
Peanuts & raisins	435	26.0
Potato Crisps	500	30.0
Potato Crisps, low fat	456	21.5
Popcorn, sugar coated	592	20.0
Desserts: per 100g		
Bread pudding	297	9.6
Cheesecake	242	10.6
Christmas pudding	329	11.8
Cream Horns	435	35.8
Custard tarts	277	14.5
Custard, made with skim milk	79	0.1
Custard, made with whole milk	117	4.5

Danish	374	17.6
Fruit pie	369	15.5
Greek cakes	322	17.0
Jam tarts	380	13.0
Jelly, fruit flavour	280	1.0
Lemon meringue pie	319	14.4
Mince pies	423	20.4
Mousse, chocolate	139	5.4
Rice pudding	89	2.5
Shortcrust pastry	449	27.9
Sponge pudding	160	3.0
Trifle	160	6.3
Wholemeal pastry	431	28.4

Soups, Sauces & Miscellaneous

Chutney: per 100g	Cal	Fat
Apple	201	0.2
Mango	285	10.9
Tomato	161	0.4
Miscellaneous		
Baking Powder	163	1.0
Gelatin	338	0
Gravy granules, made with water	325	1.0
Mustard, smooth	139	8.2
Mustard, wholegrain	140	10.2
Oxo Cubes	229	3.4
Salt	0	0
Vinegar	4	0
Pickle: per 100g		
Sweet	134	0.3
Salad Dressing: per 100g		
French dressing	649	72.1
Mayonnaise	691	75.6

Sauce: per 100g

Barbecue	75	1.8
Cheese sauce, made with skim milk	179	12.6
Cook-in sauces, canned, average	43	0.8
Mint sauce	87	1.0
Pasta sauce, tomato based	47	1.5
Soy sauce	64	0
Tomato ketchup	98	1.0
Tomato sauce, home-made	89	5.5

Soup: per 100g

Chicken noodle, dried	20	0.3
Cream of chicken, canned	58	3.8
Cream of mushroom, canned	53	3.8
Cream of tomato, canned	55	3.3
Instant soup powder (average)	64	2.3
Low calorie (average)	20	0.2
Minestrone	298	8.8
Vegetable, canned	37	0.7

Sugar, Syrups & Preservatives

Preserves: per 100g	Cal	Fat
Jam, fruit	261	0
Jam, stone fruit	261	0
Jam, reduced sugar	123	0
Lemon curd	283	5.1
Marmalade	261	0
Spreads: per 100g		
Chocolate nut	549	33.0
Honey	288	0
Syrups: per 100g		
Treacle	257	0
Golden Syrup	298	0

Fats & Oils

Butter (average all brands)	Cal	Fat
Butter	737	81.7
Low fat spread	390	40.5
Margarine	739	81.6
Margarine, polyunsaturated	739	81.6
Oils (average all brands)		
Vegetable Oil (per 20ml)	176	20.0
Fish Oil (per 20ml)	170	19.0
Oil Sprays e.g.Canola (per 20g)	140	16.0

Alcoholic Drinks

Ale: per 100ml	Cal	Fat
Bottled, brown	28	0
Bottled, pale	32	0
Strong	72	0
Beer: per 100ml		
Bitter, canned	32	0
Bitter, draught	32	0
Bitter, keg	31	0
Mild, draught	25	0
Stout	37	0
Stout, extra	39	0
Cider: per 100ml		
Dry	36	0
Sweet	42	0
Vintage	101	0
Fortified Wine: per 30ml		
Port,	47	0
Sherry, dry	35	0
Sherry, medium	35	0
Sherry, sweet	43	0

Spirits: per 30ml		
Brandy	65	0
Gin	65	0
Rum	65	0
Vodka	65	0
Whisky	65	0
Wine: per 100ml		
Red	68	0
Rose, medium	71	0
White, dry	66	0
White, medium	75	0
White, sparkling	76	0
White, sweet	94	0
Non-Alcoholic beverages: per 100g		
Carbonated drink		
Coca-cola	36	0
Lemonade	21	0
Lucozade, bottled	69	0
Cocoa		
Semi skimmed milk	57	1.9
Whole milk	76	4.2
Powder	312	21.7
Coffee		
Instant	450	0
Powder	540	34.9

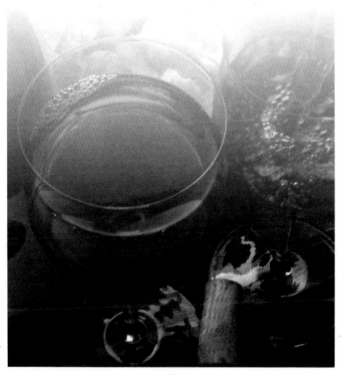

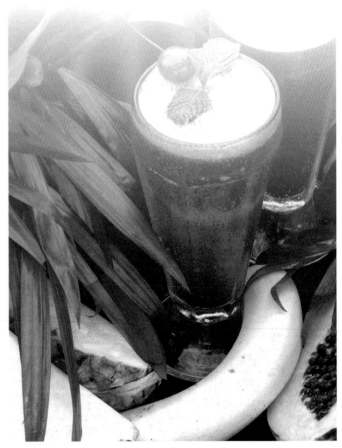

Juice

	Cal	Fat
Apple juice, unsweetened	38	0.1
Grape juice, unsweetened	46	0.1
Grapefruit juice, unsweetened	33	0.1
Lemon juice, unsweetened	07	1.0
Orange juice, unsweetened	36	0.1
Pineapple juice, unsweetened	41	0.1
Tomato juice	14	1.0
Tea		
No milk or sugar	01	1.0

Notes